THE EASIEST ANTI-INFLAMMATORY DIET 2021

Contents

Introduction

Chapter one

Fast facts on arthritis

Types

    Inflammatory arthritis

    Degenerative or mechanical arthritis

    Soft tissue musculoskeletal pain

    Back pain

    Connective tissue disease (CTD)

    Infectious arthritis

    Metabolic arthritis

Others include;

    Rheumatoid arthritis

    Osteoarthritis

    Childhood arthritis

    Septic arthritis

    Fibromyalgia

    Psoriatic arthritis

    Gout

Sjögren's syndrome

Early signs

Causes

Risk factors for arthritis

Non-modifiable arthritis risk factors:

Modifiable arthritis risk factors:

Comorbidities

Diagnosis

Treatment

Medication

Natural remedies

Diet

Self-management

Seven habits that can help a person with arthritis to manage their condition are:

Being organized:

Managing pain and fatigue:

Staying active:

Balancing activity with rest:

Eating a healthful diet:

Improving sleep:

Caring for joints:

Physical therapies

Warm water therapy:

Physical therapy:

Occupational therapy:

- Physical activity
- Natural therapies
- Surgery

What lifestyle changes can help people with arthritis?
- Food to eat
- Foods to avoid

Chapter two

Diet recipes

Turmeric Chicken & Quinoa
- Ingredients
- Instructions
- Nutrition

Anti Inflammatory Buddha Bowl
- Ingredients
- Directions

Cherry Mango Smoothie.
- Ingredients
- Instructions
- Nutrition Facts

Cannellini Beans with Garlic and Sage
- INGREDIENTS
- RECIPE PREPARATION

Lemon Basil Baked Garlic Butter Salmon

    Ingredients

    Instructions

    Nutrition

Green Papaya Salad

    Ingredients

    Directions

    Nutrition Facts

Thai Pumpkin Soup

    Ingredients

    Instructions

Mediterranean Tuna Salad

    Ingredients

    Directions

Slow Cooker Turkey Chili

    Ingredients

    Instructions

GINGERBREAD OATMEAL RECIPE:

    Ingredients

    Instructions

    Nutrition Facts

Kale Cesar Salad with Grilled Chicken Wrap

    Ingredients

    Instructions

THE BAKED TILAPIA RECIPE:

Ingredients

Instructions

Nutrition

WINTER FRUIT SALAD WITH PERSIMMONS, PEARS, GRAPES, AND PECANS

INGREDIENTS:

DRESSING INGREDIENTS:

DIRECTIONS:

Roasted Red Pepper and Sweet Potato Soup

Ingredients

Instructions

ONE PAN LEMON HERB SALMON AND ZUCCHINI

INGREDIENTS:

FOR THE SALMON

DIRECTIONS:

Smoked Salmon Potato Tartine

INGREDIENTS

POTATO TARTINE:

TOPPINGS:

INSTRUCTIONS

NUTRITION INFORMATION:

Red Lentil and Squash Curry Stew

Ingredients:

    Directions

Turkey & Quinoa Stuffed Peppers

    Ingredients:

    Directions:

Chapter three

Conclusion

Introduction

Arthritis is an inflammation of the joints. It can affect one joint or multiple joints. There are more than 100 different types of arthritis, with different causes and treatment methods. Two of the most common types are osteoarthritis (OA) and rheumatoid arthritis (RA).

The symptoms of arthritis usually develop over time, but they may also appear suddenly. Arthritis is most commonly seen in adults over the age of 65, but it can also develop in children, teens, and younger adults. Arthritis is more common in women than men and in people who are overweight.

Chapter one

Arthritis means joint inflammation, but the term is used to describe around 200 conditions that affect joints, the tissues that surround the joint, and other connective tissue. It is a rheumatic condition.

The most common form of arthritis is osteoarthritis. Other common rheumatic conditions related to arthritis include gout, fibromyalgia, and rheumatoid arthritis (RA).

Rheumatic conditions tend to involve pain, aching, stiffness, and swelling in and around one or more joints. The symptoms can develop gradually or suddenly. Certain rheumatic conditions can also involve the immune system and various internal organs of the body.

Some forms of arthritis, such as rheumatoid arthritis and lupus (SLE), can affect multiple organs and cause widespread symptoms.

According to the Centers for Disease Control and Prevention (CDC), 54.4 million adults in the United States have received a diagnosis of some form of arthritis. Of these, 23.7 million people have their activity curtailed in some way by their condition.

Arthritis is more common among adults aged 65 years or older, but it can affect people of all ages, including children.

Fast facts on arthritis

Arthritis refers to around 200 rheumatic diseases and conditions that affect joints, including lupus and rheumatoid arthritis.

It can cause a range of symptoms and impair a person's ability to perform everyday tasks.

Physical activity has a positive effect on arthritis and can improve pain, function, and mental health.

Factors in the development of arthritis include injury, abnormal metabolism, genetic makeup, infections, and immune system dysfunction.

Treatment aims to control pain, minimize joint damage, and improve or maintain quality of life. It involves medications, physical therapies, and patient education and support.

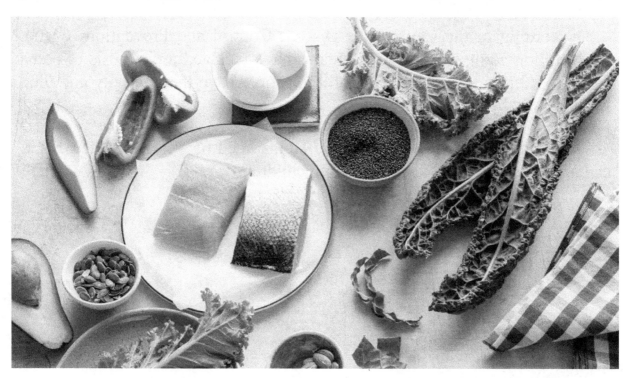

Types

There are around 200 types of arthritis, or musculoskeletal conditions. These are split into seven main groups:

Inflammatory arthritis

Degenerative or mechanical arthritis

Soft tissue musculoskeletal pain

Back pain

Connective tissue disease

Infectious arthritis

Metabolic arthritis.

Inflammatory arthritis

Inflammatory arthritis

Inflammation is a normal part of the body's healing process. The inflammation tends to occur as a defense against viruses and bacteria or as a response to injuries such as burns. However, with inflammatory arthritis, inflammation occurs in people for no apparent reason.

Inflammatory arthritis can affect several joints, damaging the surface of the joints and the underlying bone.

Inflammatory arthritis is characterized by damaging inflammation that does not occur as a normal reaction to injury or infection. This type of inflammation is unhelpful and instead causes damage in the affected joints, resulting in pain, stiffness and swelling.

Inflammatory arthritis can affect several joints, and the inflammation can damage the surface of the joints and also the underlying bone.

Examples of inflammatory arthritis include:

Rheumatoid arthritis (RA)

Reactive arthritis

Ankylosing spondylitis

Arthritis associated with colitis or psoriasis

The word "arthritis" means "joint inflammation," but inflammation may also affect the tendons and ligaments surrounding the joint.

Degenerative or mechanical arthritis

Degenerative or mechanical arthritis refers to a group of conditions that mainly involve damage to the cartilage that covers the ends of the bones.

The main job of the smooth, slippery cartilage is to help the joints glide and move smoothly. This type of arthritis causes the cartilage to become thinner and rougher.

To compensate for the loss of cartilage and changes in joint function, the body begins to remodel the bone in an attempt to restore stability. This can cause undesirable bony growths to develop, called osteophytes. The joint can become misshapen. This condition is commonly called osteoarthritis.

Osteoarthritis can also result from previous damage to the joint such as a fracture or previous inflammation in the joint.

Soft tissue musculoskeletal pain

Soft tissue musculoskeletal pain is felt in tissues other than the joints and bones. The pain often affects a part of the body following injury or overuse, such as tennis elbow, and originates from the muscles or soft tissues supporting the joints.

Pain that is more widespread and associated with other symptoms may indicate fibromyalgia.

Back pain

Back pain can arise from the muscles, discs, nerves, ligaments, bones, or joints. Back pain may stem from problems with organs inside the body. It can also be a result of referred pain, for example, when a problem elsewhere in the body leads to pain in the back.

There may be a specific cause, such as osteoarthritis. This is often called spondylosis when it occurs in the spine. Imaging tests or a physical examination may detect this.

Connective tissue disease (CTD)

Connective tissues support, bind together, or separate other body tissues and organs. They include tendons, ligaments, and cartilage.

CTD involves joint pain and inflammation. The inflammation may also occur in other tissues, including the skin, muscles, lungs, and kidneys. This can result in various symptoms besides painful joints, and it may require consultation with a number of different specialists.

Examples of CTD include:

SLE, or lupus

Scleroderma, or systemic sclerosis

dermatomyositis.

Infectious arthritis

A bacterium, virus, or fungus that enters a joint can sometimes cause inflammation.

Organisms that can infect joints include:

Salmonella and Shigella, spread through food poisoning or contamination

Chlamydia and gonorrhea, which are sexually transmitted diseases (STDs)

Hepatitis C, a blood-to-blood infection that may be spread through shared needles or transfusions

A joint infection can often be cleared with antibiotics or other antimicrobial medication. However, the arthritis can sometimes become chronic, and joint damage may be irreversible if the infection has persisted for some time.

Metabolic arthritis

Uric acid is a chemical created when the body breaks down substances called purines. Purines are found in human cells and several foods.

Most uric acid dissolves in blood and travels to the kidneys. From there, it passes out in urine. Some people have high levels of uric, acid because they either naturally produce more than they need or their body cannot clear the uric acid quickly enough.

Uric acid builds up and accumulates in some people and forms needle-like crystals in the joint, resulting in sudden spikes of extreme joint pain or a gout attack.

Gout can either come and go in episodes or become chronic if uric acid levels are not reduced.

It commonly affects a single joint or a small number of joints, such as the big toe and hands. It usually affects the extremities. One theory is that uric acid crystals form in cooler joints, away from the main warmth of the body.

Others include;

Some of the more common types of arthritis are discussed below.

Rheumatoid arthritis

Rheumatoid arthritis and osteoarthritis share some characteristics, but they are different conditions.

Rheumatoid arthritis (RA) occurs when the body's immune system attacks the tissues of the body, specifically connective tissue, leading to joint inflammation, pain, and degeneration of the joint tissue.

Cartilage is a flexible, connective tissue in joints that absorb the pressure and shock created by movement like running and walking. It also protects the joints and allows for smooth movement.

Persistent inflammation in the synovia leads to the degeneration of cartilage and bone. This can then lead to joint deformity, pain, swelling, and redness.

RA can appear at any age and is associated with fatigue and prolonged stiffness after rest.

RA causes premature mortality and disability and it can compromise quality of life. Conditions it is linked to include cardiovascular diseases, such as ischemic heart disease and stroke.

Diagnosing RA early gives a better chance of learning how to manage symptoms successfully. This can reduce the impact of the disease on quality of life.

Osteoarthritis

Osteoarthritis is caused by a reduction in the normal amount of cartilage tissue through wear and tear throughout life.

Osteoarthritis is a common degenerative joint disease that affects the cartilage, joint lining and ligaments, and underlying bone of a joint.

The breakdown of these tissues eventually leads to pain and joint stiffness.

The joints most often affected by osteoarthritis are those that get heavy use, such as hips, knees, hands, the spine, the base of the thumb, and the big toe joint.

Childhood arthritis

This can refer to a number of types of arthritis. Juvenile idiopathic arthritis (JIA), also known as juvenile rheumatoid arthritis (JRA), is the most common type.

Arthritis in childhood can cause permanent damage to joints, and there is no cure. However, remission is possible, during which time the disease remains inactive.

It may be due to immune system problems.

Septic arthritis

This is thought to affect between 2 and 10 people in every 100,000 in the general population. Among people with RA, it may affect 30 to 70 people per 100,000.

Septic arthritis is a joint inflammation that results from a bacterial or fungal infection. It commonly affects the knee and hip.

It can develop when bacteria or other disease-causing micro-organisms spread through the blood to a joint, or when the joint is directly infected with a microorganism through injury or surgery.

Bacteria such as Staphylococcus, Streptococcus, or Neisseria gonorrhoeae cause most cases of acute septic arthritis. Organisms such as Mycobacterium tuberculosis and Candida albicans cause chronic septic arthritis. This is less common than acute septic arthritis.

Septic arthritis may occur at any age. In infants, it may occur before the age of 3 years. The hip is a common site of infection at this age.

Septic arthritis is uncommon from 3 years to adolescence. Children with septic arthritis are more likely than adults to be infected with Group B Streptococcus or Haemophilus influenzae if they have not been vaccinated.

The incidence of bacterial arthritis caused by infection with H. influenzae has decreased by around 70 percent to 80 percent since the use of the H. influenzae b (Hib) vaccine became common.

The following conditions increase the risk of developing septic arthritis:

Existing joint disease or damage

Artificial joint implants

Bacterial infection elsewhere in the body

Presence of bacteria in the blood

Chronic illness or disease (such as diabetes, RA and sickle cell disease)

Intravenous (IV) or injection drug use

Medications that suppress the immune system

Recent joint injury

Recent joint arthroscopy or other surgery

Conditions such as HIV, that weaken immunity

Diabetes

Older age

Septic arthritis is a rheumatologic emergency as it can lead to rapid joint destruction. It can be fatal.

Fibromyalgia

Fibromyalgia affects an estimated 4 million adults in the U.S, or around 2 percent of the population.

It usually starts during middle age or after, but it can affect children.

Fibromyalgia can involve:

Widespread pain

Sleep disturbance

Fatigue

Depression

Problems with thinking and remembering

The person may experience abnormal pain processing, where they reacts strongly to something that other people would not find painful.

There may also be tingling or numbness in the hands and feet, pain in the jaw, and digestive problems.

The causes of fibromyalgia are unknown, but some factors have been loosely associated with disease onset:

Stressful or traumatic events

Post-traumatic stress disorder (PTSD)

Injuries due to repetitive movements

Illness, for example viral infections

Having lupus, RA, or chronic fatigue syndrome

Family history

Obesity

It is more common among females.

Psoriatic arthritis

Psoriatic arthritis is a joint problem that often occurs with a skin condition called psoriasis. It is thought to affect between 0.3 and 1 percent of the population in the U.S., and between 6 and 42 percent of people with psoriasis.

Most people who have psoriatic arthritis and psoriasis develop psoriasis first and then psoriatic arthritis, but joint problems can occasionally occur before skin lesions appear.

The exact cause of psoriatic arthritis is not known, but it appears to involve the immune system attacking healthy cells and tissue. The abnormal immune response causes inflammation in the joints and an overproduction of skin cells. Damage to the joints can result.

Factors that increase the risk, include:

Having psoriasis

Family history

Being aged from 30 to 50 year

People with psoriatic arthritis tend to have a higher number of risk factors for cardiovascular disease than the general population, including increased BMI, triglycerides, and C-reactive protein.

Gout

Gout is a rheumatic disease that happens when uric acid crystals, or monosodium urate, form in body tissues and fluids. It happens when the body produces too much uric acid or does not excrete enough uric acid.

Gout causes agonizing pain in the joint, with the area becoming red, hot and swollen.

Acute gout normally appears as a severely red, hot, and swollen joint and severe pain.

Sjögren's syndrome

Sjögren's syndrome is an autoimmune disorder that sometimes occurs alongside RA and SLE. It involves the destruction of glands that produce tears and saliva. This causes dryness in the mouth and eyes and in other areas that usually need moisture, such as the nose, throat, and skin.

It can also affect the joints, lungs, kidneys, blood vessels, digestive organs, and nerves.

Sjögren's syndrome typically affects in adults aged 40 to 50 years, and especially women.

According to a study in Clinical and Experimental Rheumatology, in 40 to 50 percent of people with primary Sjögren's syndrome, the condition affects tissues other than the glands.

It could affect the lungs, liver, or kidneys, or it could lead to skin vasculitis, peripheral neuropathy, glomerulonephritis, and low levels of a substance known as C4. These all indicate a link between Sjögren's and the immune system.

If these tissues are affected, there is a high risk of developing non-Hodgkin's lymphoma.

Scleroderma

Scleroderma refers to a group of diseases that affect connective tissue in the body. The person will have patches of hard, dry skin. Some types can affect the internal organs and small arteries.

Scar-like tissue builds up in the skin and causes damage.

The cause is currently unknown. It often affects people between the ages of 30 to 50 years, and it may occur with other autoimmune diseases, such as lupus.

Scleroderma affects individuals differently. The complications include skin problems, weakness in the heart, lung damage, gastrointestinal problems, and kidney failure.

Systemic lupus erythematosus (SLE)

SLE, commonly known as lupus, is an autoimmune disease where the immune system produces antibodies to cells within the body leading to widespread inflammation and tissue damage. The disease is characterized by periods of illness and remissions.

It can appear at any age, but onset is most likely is between the ages of 15 and 45 years. For every one man who gets lupus, between 4 and 12 women will do so.

Lupus can affect the joints, skin, brain, lungs, kidneys, blood vessels, and other tissues. Symptoms include fatigue, pain or swelling in joints, skin rashes, and fevers.

The cause remains unclear, but it could be linked to genetic, environmental, and hormonal factors.

Early signs

The symptoms of arthritis that appear and how they appear vary widely, depending on the type.

Warning signs of arthritis include pain, swelling, stiffness and difficulty moving a joint.

They can develop gradually or suddenly. As arthritis is most often a chronic disease, symptoms may come and go, or persist over time.

However, anyone who experiences any of the following four key warning signs should see a doctor.

Pain: Pain from arthritis can be constant, or it may come and go. It may affect only one part, or be felt in many parts of the body

Swelling: In some types of arthritis the skin over the affected joint becomes red and swollen and feels warm to the touch

Stiffness. Stiffness is a typical symptom. With some types, this is most likely upon waking up in the morning, after sitting at a desk, or after sitting in a car for a long time. With other types, stiffness may occur after exercise, or it may be persistent.

Difficulty moving a joint: If moving a joint or getting up from a chair is hard or painful, this could indicate arthritis or another joint problem.

Rheumatoid arthritis

RA is a systemic disease, so it usually affects the joints on both sides of the body equally. The joints of the wrists, fingers, knees, feet and ankles are the most commonly affected.

Joint symptoms may include:

Morning stiffness, lasting more than 1 hour

Pain, often in the same joints on both sides of the body

Loss of range of motion of joints, possibly with deformity

Other symptoms include:

Chest pain when breathing in, due to pleurisy

Dry eyes and mouth, if Sjögren's syndrome is present

Eye burning, itching, and discharge

Nodules under the skin, usually a sign of more severe disease

Numbness, tingling, or burning in the hands and feet

Sleep difficulties

Osteoarthritis

Osteoarthritis is usually a result of wear and tear on the joints. It will affect joints that have been overworked more than others. People with osteoarthritis may experience the following symptoms:

Pain and stiffness in the joints

Pain that becomes worse after exercise or pressure on the joint

Rubbing, grating, or crackling sound when a joint is moved

Morning stiffness

Pain that causes sleep disturbances

Some people may have changes linked to osteoarthritis that show up in an x-ray, but they do not experience symptoms.

Osteoarthritis typically affects some joints more than others, such as the left or right knee, shoulder or wrist.

Childhood arthritis

Symptoms of childhood arthritis include:

A joint that is swollen, red, or warm

A joint that is stiff or limited in movement

Limping or difficulty using an arm or leg

A sudden high fever that may come and go

A rash on the trunk and extremities that comes and goes with the fever

Symptoms throughout the body, such as pale skin, swollen lymph glands

Generally appearing unwell

Juvenile RA can also cause eye problems including uveitis, iridocyclitis, or iritis. If eye symptoms do occur they can include:

Red eyes

Eye pain, especially when looking at light

Vision changes.

Septic arthritis

Symptoms of septic arthritis occur rapidly.

There is often:

Fever

Intense joint pain that becomes more severe with movement

Joint swelling in one joint

Symptoms in newborns or infants include:

Crying when the infected joint is moved

Fever

Inability to move the limb with the infected joint

Irritability

Symptoms in children and adults include:

Inability to move the limb with the infected joint

Intense joint pain, swelling, and redness

Fever.

Chills sometimes occur but are an uncommon symptom.

Fibromyalgia

Fibromyalgia may trigger the following symptoms:

Fibromyalgia has many symptoms that tend to vary from person to person. The main symptom is widespread pain.

- Widespread pain, often with specific tender points
- Sleep disturbance
- Fatigue
- Psychological stress
- Morning stiffness
- Tingling or numbness in hands and feet
- Headaches, including migraines
- Irritable bowel syndrome
- Problems with thinking and memory, sometimes called "fibro fog"
- Painful menstrual periods and other pain syndromes

Psoriatic arthritis

Symptoms of psoriatic arthritis may be mild and involve only a few joints such as the end of the fingers or toes.

Severe psoriatic arthritis can affect multiple joints, including the spine. Spinal symptoms are usually felt in the lower spine and sacrum. These consist of stiffness, burning, and pain.

People with psoriatic arthritis often have the skin and nail changes of psoriasis, and the skin gets worse at the same time as the arthritis.

Gout

Symptoms of gout involve:

Pain and swelling, often in the big toe, knee, or ankle joints

Sudden pain, often during the night, which may be throbbing, crushing, or excruciating

Warm and tender joints that appear red and swollen

Fever sometimes occurs

After having gout for many years, a person can develop tophi. Tophi are lumps below the skin, typically around the joints or apparent on fingertips and ears. Multiple, small tophi may develop, or a large white lump. This can cause deformation and stretching of the skin.

Sometimes, tophi burst and drain spontaneously, oozing a white, chalky substance. Tophi that are beginning to break through the skin can lead to infection or osteomyelitis. Some patients will need urgent surgery to drain the tophus.

Sjögren's syndrome

Symptoms of Sjögren's syndrome include:

Dry and itchy eyes, and a feeling that something is in the eye

Dry mouth

Difficulty swallowing or eating

Loss of sense of taste

Problems speaking

Thick or stringy saliva

Mouth sores or pain

Hoarseness

Fatigue

Fever

Change in color of hands or feet

Joint pain or joint swelling

Swollen glands

Scleroderma

Symptoms of scleroderma may include:

Fingers or toes that turn blue or white in response to cold temperatures, known as Raynaud's phenomenon

Hair loss

Skin that becomes darker or lighter than normal

Stiffness and tightness of skin on the fingers, hands, forearm, and face

Small white lumps beneath the skin that sometimes ooze a white substance that looks like toothpaste

Sores or ulcers on the fingertips or toes

Tight and mask-like skin on the face

Numbness and pain in the feet

Pain, stiffness, and swelling of the wrist, fingers, and other joints

Dry cough, shortness of breath, and wheezing

Gastrointestinal problems, such as bloating after meals, constipation, and diarrhea

Difficulty swallowing

Esophageal reflux or heartburn

Systemic lupus erythematosus (SLE)

The most common signs of SLE, or lupus, are:

Red rash or color change on the face, often in the shape of a butterfly across the nose and cheeks

Painful or swollen joints

Unexplained fever

Chest pain when breathing deeply

Swollen glands

Extreme fatigue

Unusual hair loss

Pale or purple fingers or toes from cold or stress

Sensitivity to the sun

Low blood count

Depression, trouble thinking or memory problems.

Other signs are mouth sores, unexplained seizures, hallucinations, repeated miscarriages, and unexplained kidney problems.

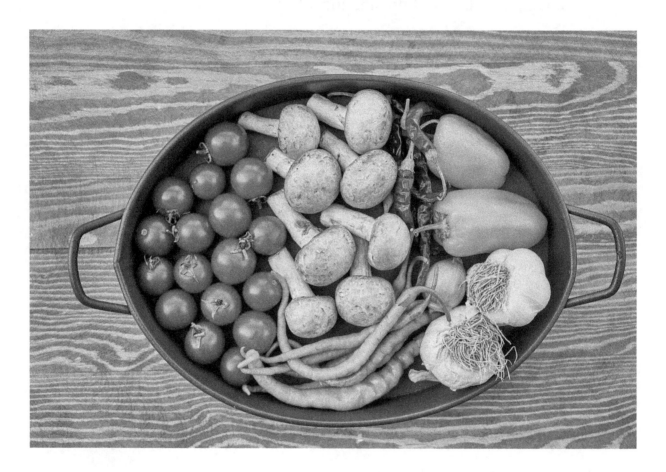

Causes

There is no single cause of all types of arthritis. The cause or causes vary according to the type or form of arthritis.

Possible causes may include:

Injury, leading to degenerative arthritis

Abnormal metabolism, leading to gout and pseudogout

Inheritance, such as in osteoarthritis

Infections, such as in the arthritis of Lyme disease

Immune system dysfunction, such as in RA and SLE

Most types of arthritis are linked to a combination of factors, but some have no obvious cause and appear to be unpredictable in their emergence.

Some people may be genetically more likely to develop certain arthritic conditions. Additional factors, such as previous injury, infection, smoking and physically demanding occupations, can interact with genes to further increase the risk of arthritis.

Diet and nutrition can play a role in managing arthritis and the risk of arthritis, although specific foods, food sensitivities or intolerances are not known to cause arthritis.

Foods that increase inflammation, particularly animal-derived foods and diets high in refined sugar, can make symptoms worse, as can eating foods that provoke an immune system response.

Gout is one type of arthritis that is closely linked to diet, as it is caused by elevated levels of uric acid which can be a result of a diet high in purines.

Diets that contain high-purine foods, such as seafood, red wine, and meats, can trigger a gout flare-up. Vegetables and other plant foods that contain high levels of purines do not appear to exacerbate gout symptoms, however.

Risk factors for arthritis

Certain risk factors have been associated with arthritis. Some of these are modifiable while others are not.

Non-modifiable arthritis risk factors:

Age: the risk of developing most types of arthritis increases with age.

Sex: most types of arthritis are more common in females, and 60 percent of all people with arthritis are female. Gout is more common in males than females.

Genetic factors: specific genes are associated with a higher risk of certain types of arthritis, such as rheumatoid arthritis (RA), systemic lupus erythematosus (SLE) and ankylosing spondylitis.

Modifiable arthritis risk factors:

Overweight and obesity: excess weight can contribute to both the onset and progression of knee osteoarthritis.

Joint injuries: damage to a joint can contribute to the development of osteoarthritis in that joint.

Infection: many microbial agents can infect joints and trigger the development of various forms of arthritis.

Occupation: certain occupations that involve repetitive knee bending and squatting are associated with osteoarthritis of the knee.

Comorbidities

More than half of adults in the U.S. with arthritis report high blood pressure. High blood pressure is associated with heart disease, the most common comorbidity among adults with arthritis.

Around 1 in 5 of adults in the U.S. who have arthritis are smokers. Smoking is associated with chronic respiratory conditions, the second most common comorbidity among adults with arthritis.

Diagnosis

Seeing your primary care physician is a good first step if you're unsure who to see for an arthritis diagnosis. They will perform a physical exam to check for fluid around the joints, warm or red joints, and limited range of motion in the joints. Your doctor can refer you to a specialist if needed.

If you're experiencing severe symptoms, you may choose to schedule an appointment with a rheumatologist first. This may lead to a faster diagnosis and treatment. Extracting and analyzing inflammation levels in your blood and joint fluids can help your doctor determine what kind of arthritis you have. Blood tests that check for specific types of antibodies like anti-CCP (anti-cyclic citrullinated peptide), RF (rheumatoid factor), and ANA (antinuclear antibody) are also common diagnostic tests.

Doctors commonly use imaging scans such as X-ray, MRI, and CT scans to produce an image of your bones and cartilage. This is so they can rule out other causes of your symptoms, such as bone spurs.

Treatment

Treatment for arthritis aims to control pain, minimize joint damage, and improve or maintain function and quality of life.

A range of medications and lifestyle strategies can help achieve this and protect joints from further damage.

Treatment might involve:

Medications

Non-pharmacologic therapies

Physical or occupational therapy

Splints or joint assistive aids

Patient education and support

Weight loss

Surgery, including joint replacement

Medication

Non-inflammatory types of arthritis, such as osteoarthritis, are often treated with pain-reducing medications, physical activity, weight loss if the person is overweight, and self-management education.

These treatments are also applied to inflammatory types of arthritis, such as RA, along with anti-inflammatory medications such as corticosteroids and non-steroidal anti-inflammatory drugs (NSAIDs), disease-modifying anti-rheumatic drugs (DMARDs), and a relatively new class of drugs known as biologics.

Medications will depend on the type of arthritis. Commonly used drugs include:

Analgesics: these reduce pain, but have no effect on inflammation. Examples include acetaminophen (Tylenol), tramadol (Ultram) and narcotics containing oxycodone (Percocet, Oxycontin) or hydrocodone (Vicodin, Lortab). Tylenol is available to purchase online.

Non-steroidal anti-inflammatory drugs (NSAIDs): these reduce both pain and inflammation. NSAIDs include available to purchase over-the-counter or online, including ibuprofen (Advil, Motrin IB) and naproxen sodium (Aleve). Some NSAIDs are available as creams, gels or patches which can be applied to specific joints.

Counterirritants: some creams and ointments contain menthol or capsaicin, the ingredient that makes hot peppers spicy. Rubbing these on the skin over a painful joint can modulate pain signals from the joint and lessen pain. Various creams are available to purchase online.

Disease-modifying antirheumatic drugs (DMARDs): used to treat RA, DMARDs slow or stop the immune system from attacking the joints. Examples include methotrexate (Trexall) and hydroxychloroquine (Plaquenil).

Biologics: used with DMARDs, biologic response modifiers are genetically engineered drugs that target various protein molecules involved in the immune response. Examples include etanercept (Enbrel) and infliximab (Remicade).

Corticosteroids: prednisone and cortisone reduce inflammation and suppress the immune system.

Natural remedies

A healthful, balanced diet with appropriate exercise, avoiding smoking, and not drinking excess alcohol can help people with arthritis maintain their overall health.

Diet

There is no specific diet that treats arthritis, but some types of food may help reduce inflammation.

The following foods, found in a Mediterranean diet, can provide many nutrients that are good for joint health:

Fish

Nuts and seeds

Fruits and vegetables

Beans

Olive oil

Whole grains

Foods to avoid

There are some foods that people with arthritis may want to avoid.

Nightshade vegetables, such as tomatoes, contain a chemical called solanine that some studies have linked with arthritis pain. Research findings are mixed when it comes to these vegetables, but some people have reported a reduction in arthritis symptoms when avoiding nightshade vegetables.

Self-management

Self-management of arthritis symptoms is also important.

Key strategies include:

Staying physically active

Achieving and maintaining a healthy weight

Getting regular check-ups with the doctor

Protecting joints from unnecessary stress

Seven habits that can help a person with arthritis to manage their condition are:

Being organized:
Keep track of symptoms, pain levels, medications, and possible side effects for consultations with your doctor.

Managing pain and fatigue:
A medication regimen can be combined with non-medical pain management. Learning to manage fatigue is key to living comfortably with arthritis.

Staying active:
Exercise is beneficial for managing arthritis and overall health.

Balancing activity with rest:
In addition to remaining active, rest is equally important when your disease is active.

Eating a healthful diet:
A balanced diet can help you achieve a healthy weight and control inflammation. Avoid refined, processed foods and pro-inflammatory animal-derived foods and choose whole plant foods that are high in antioxidants and that have anti-inflammatory properties.

Improving sleep:
poor sleep can aggravate arthritis pain and fatigue. Take steps to improve sleep hygiene so you find it easier to fall asleep and stay asleep. Avoid caffeine and strenuous exercise in the evenings and restrict screen-time just before sleeping.

Caring for joints:
Tips for protecting joints include using the stronger, larger joints as levers when opening doors, using several joints to spread the weight of an object such as using a backpack and gripping as loosely as possible by using padded handles.

Do not sit in the same position for long periods. Take regular breaks to keep mobile.

Physical therapies
Doctors will often recommend a course of physical therapy to help patients with arthritis overcome some of the challenges and to reduce limitations on mobility.

Forms of physical therapy that may be recommended include:

Warm water therapy:
Exercises in a warm-water pool. The water supports weight and puts less pressure on the muscles and joints

Physical therapy:
Specific exercises tailored to the condition and individual needs, sometimes combined with pain-relieving treatments such as ice or hot packs and massage

Occupational therapy:
Practical advice on managing everyday tasks, choosing specialized aids and equipment, protecting the joints from further damage and managing fatigue

Physical activity
Research suggests that although individuals with arthritis may experience short-term increases in pain when first beginning exercise, continued physical activity can be an effective way to reduce symptoms long-term.

People with arthritis can participate in joint-friendly physical activity on their own or with friends. As many people with arthritis have another condition, such as heart disease, it is important to choose appropriate activities.

Joint-friendly physical activities that are appropriate for adults with arthritis and heart disease include:

Walking

Swimming

Cycling

A health care professional can help you find ways to live a healthful lifestyle and have a better quality of life.

Natural therapies

A number of natural remedies have been suggested for different types of arthritis.

According to the organization Versus Arthritis, based in the United Kingdom (U.K.), some research has supported the use of devil's claw, rosehip, and Boswellia, from the frankincense tree. Devil's claw and Boswellia supplements can be purchased online.

There is some evidence that turmeric may help, but more studies are needed to confirm their effectiveness.

Various other herbs and spices have been recommended for RA, but again, more research is needed. They include turmeric, garlic, ginger, black pepper, and green tea.

Many of these herbs and spices are available to purchase online in supplement form, including turmeric, ginger, and garlic.

Surgery

Surgery to replace your joint with an artificial one may be an option. This form of surgery is most commonly performed to replace hips and knees.

If your arthritis is most severe in your fingers or wrists, your doctor may perform a joint fusion. In this procedure, the ends of your bones are locked together until they heal and become one.

What lifestyle changes can help people with arthritis?

Weight loss and maintaining a healthy weight reduce the risk of developing OA and can reduce symptoms if you already have it.

Eating a healthy diet is important for weight loss. Choosing a diet with lots of antioxidants, such as fresh fruits, vegetables, and herbs, can help reduce inflammation. Other inflammation-reducing foods include fish and nuts.

Foods to minimize or avoid if you have arthritis include fried foods, processed foods, dairy products, and high intakes of meat.

Some research also suggests that gluten antibodies may be present in people with RA. A gluten-free diet may improve symptoms and disease progression. A 2015 study also recommends a gluten-free diet for all people who receive a diagnosis of undifferentiated connective tissue disease.

Regular exercise will keep your joints flexible. Swimming is often a good form of exercise for people with arthritis because it doesn't put pressure on your joints the way running and walking do. Staying active is important, but you should also be sure to rest when you need to and avoid overexerting yourself.

At-home exercises you can try include:

The head tilt, neck rotation, and other exercises to relieve pain in your neck

Finger bends and thumb bends to ease pain in your hands

Leg raises, hamstring stretches, and other easy exercises for knee arthritis

Food to eat

List of key foods to include

Cooking with olive oil may help relieve inflammation.

According to the Arthritis Foundation, around two-thirds of a person's diet should come from whole grains, fruits, and vegetables. The remaining one-third should comprise low-fat dairy and lean protein sources.

Some of the foods that research has shown to relieve inflammation include cold-water fish that contain omega-3 fatty acids. Examples of these fish include:

Herring

Mackerel

Salmon

Trout

Tuna

Extra-virgin olive oil could also help fight inflammation. Many doctors recommend creating recipes from a Mediterranean diet, which is usually rich in fish, fruits, vegetables, and whole grains.

Foods rich in vitamin D may also help reduce inflammation. Examples include:

Cereals fortified with vitamin D

Eggs

Fortified bread

Low-fat milk fortified with vitamin D

Mushrooms

Foods to avoid

Just as some foods appear to fight inflammation, others may increase it.

Fried foods can increase the number of compounds called advanced glycation end products (AGEs) in a person's blood. The levels of AGEs tend to be high in people with inflammation, so it is likely that they play a role in its development.

Excess omega-6 fatty acids may also cause inflammation if a person does not have enough anti-inflammatory omega-3 fatty acids in their diet to balance them out.

Sources of omega-6 fatty acids include some cooking oils, such as corn, sunflower, safflower, and soybean oils.

Chapter two

Diet recipes

Turmeric Chicken & Quinoa

Prep Time 20 mins

Cook Time 56 mins

Total Time 1 hr 16 mins

Ingredients

2 pounds boneless skinless chicken or tempeh

1 teaspoon salt

1/2 teaspoon fresh ground black pepper

1 tablespoon extra virgin olive oil

1 teaspoon ground turmeric

1 onion chopped

1 tablespoon grated chopped peeled fresh ginger

4 cloves garlic minced

2 plum tomatoes chopped

1 1/2 teaspoon curry powder

1/2 teaspoon ground cumin

2 cups quinoa rinsed

2 bay leaves

1 1/2 tablespoons Asian fish sauce

2 3/4 cups chicken broth or vegetable broth

Instructions

Season the chicken with salt and pepper. In a large Dutch Oven, heat the olive oil to medium and add turmeric. Stir and add chicken.

Cook until browned on both sides. Transfer to a plate. Allow to cool and then shred.

Add the onion and ginger and cook for 8 minutes. Add garlic, tomatoes, curry powder, cumin and quinoa. Cook, string constantly for 3 minutes.

Return the chicken to the pot. Add bay leaves, fish sauce and chicken broth. Bring to a simmer.

Cover and cook over low heat for 25 minutes. Remove from heat and let stand covered for 5 minutes.

Nutrition

Calories: 320kcal | Carbohydrates: 30g | Protein: 31g | Fat: 7g | Saturated Fat: 1g | Cholesterol: 72mg | Sodium: 987mg | Potassium: 808mg | Fiber: 3g | Sugar: 1g | Vitamin A: 165IU | Vitamin C: 10.6mg | Calcium: 41mg | Iron: 3mg

Anti Inflammatory Buddha Bowl

Makes 4 servings

Ingredients

2lb cauliflower florets, steams removed and broken into chunks

1 TBSP extra virgin olive oil

1 tsp. turmeric

Salt and pepper

10oz chopped kale

1 clove of garlic

8 medium cooked beets, peeled and quartered

2 avocados

2c blueberries

1/3c chopped raw walnuts

Optional ingredients, cayenne pepper and nutritional yeast.

Directions

Preheat oven to 425F. Line a rimmed baking sheet with foil, spray with coconut or olive oil and set aside. In a large bowl toss cauliflower with olive oil. Sprinkle in turmeric and toss. Spread cauliflower on baking sheet and wash your hands. Sprinkle generously with sea salt and pepper as well as a little cayenne pepper and nutritional yeast if desired. Bake cauliflower for about 30 minutes, checking at 20 minutes. When your cauliflower is just about done heat a large skillet or fry pan with a little coconut oil spray or a small drizzle of oil over medium heat. Add in kale and toss until it just starts to wilt and grate in garlic. Toss to coat. I don't like mushy kale but you can cook it longer if desired. Cut avocado into chunks or slices. Divide kale among bowls, top with roasted turmeric cauliflower, beets, avocado, blueberries, and walnuts. Enjoy!

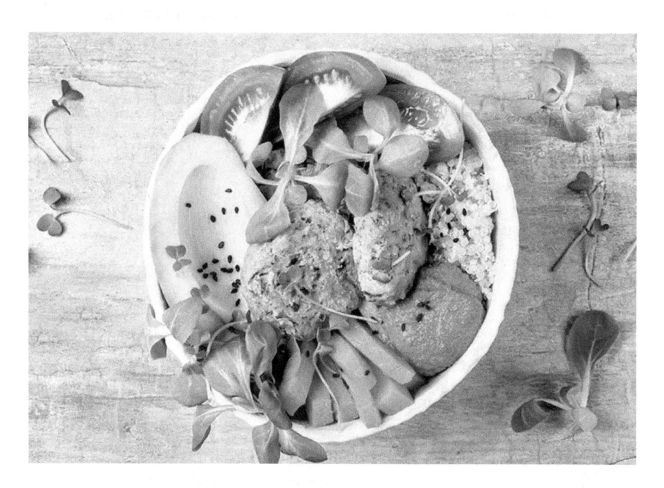

Cherry Mango Smoothie.

Prep Time 10 minutes

Cook Time 5 minutes

Total Time 15 minutes

Servings 1

Ingredients

1 cup frozen sweet cherries

1/2 cup water

1 cup frozen mango

3/4 cup water

Instructions

Place the cherries and mangoes in two separate bowls and let them sit to thaw for about ten minutes.

Blend the cherries first: place the cherries and a 1/2 cup water in the blender and blend on high until smooth. Add the other 1/4 cup water if it seems too thick. Pour into a glass.

Rinse the blender pitcher and add the mango and the water. Blend on high until smooth. Add more water if needed. Pour into the glass on top of the cherry layer.

Nutrition Facts

Cherry Mango Anti-Inflammatory Smoothie.

Amount Per Serving

Calories 185

% Daily Value*

Sodium 17mg 1%

Potassium 583mg 17%

Carbohydrates 46g 15%

Fiber 5g 21%

Sugar 40g 44%

Protein 2g 4%

Vitamin A 1875IU 38%

Vitamin C 69.7mg 84%

Calcium 36mg 4%

Iron 0.8mg 4%

* Percent Daily Values are based on a 2000 calorie diet.

Cannellini Beans with Garlic and Sage

INGREDIENTS

1 pound dried cannellini (white kidney beans)

8 cups room-temperature water

2 tablespoons olive oil

1 large head of garlic, unpeeled, top 1/2 inch cut off to expose cloves

1 large fresh sage sprig

1/4 teaspoon whole black peppercorns

1 teaspoon coarse kosher salt

Extra-virgin olive oil (for drizzling)

RECIPE PREPARATION

Place beans in large bowl. Cover with cold water (at least 6 cups) and let soak overnight.

Drain beans. Place in heavy large pot. Add 8 cups room-temperature water, 2 tablespoons olive oil, garlic, sage, and black peppercorns. Bring to simmer over medium-high heat. Reduce heat to medium-low; simmer uncovered 1 1/2 hours, stirring occasionally. Mix in 1 teaspoon coarse salt. Continue to simmer until beans are tender, adding more water if needed to keep beans covered, about 30 minutes longer. Cool beans in liquid 1 hour.

Using slotted spoon, transfer beans to serving bowl, reserving bean cooking liquid, if desired, but discarding garlic, sage, and peppercorns.

Season beans to taste with pepper and more coarse salt. Drizzle with extra-virgin olive oil and serve.

Lemon Basil Baked Garlic Butter Salmon

Prep Time: 5 minutes Cook Time: 18 minutes Total Time: 23 minutes
Servings: 4Calories: 285kcal

Ingredients

6 ounces salmon (4 pieces)

2 lemons

1/2 cup butter

2 Tbs minced garlic

1 tsp sweet basil leaf dried

1 pinch red pepper flakes more if you like it spicy

1 spray PAM cooking spray

Instructions

Preheat oven to 375 degrees F.

Lay out your foil sheets, one per filet of fish.

Put your salmon on your foil.

In a microwave safe bowl, combine butter, garlic, basil, and red pepper.

Microwave 30 seconds to 1 minute until butter is melted, stir well.

Spoon butter mixture evenly over the fish

Squeeze half a lemon over each filet

Wrap in foil, place on baking sheet

Bake for 15-17 minutes, until desired doneness is reached

Turn oven on to broil on high

Broil 1-2 minutes to crisp up edges of Salmon

Serve immediately.

Nutrition

Calories: 285kcal | Carbohydrates: 6g | Protein: 9g | Fat: 25g | Saturated Fat: 15g | Cholesterol: 84mg | Sodium: 223mg | Potassium: 298mg | Fiber: 1g | Sugar: 1g | Vitamin A: 725IU | Vitamin C: 29.9mg | Calcium: 33mg | Iron: 0.7mg

Green Papaya Salad

Total: 35 mins

Servings: 6

Ingredients

¼ teaspoon freshly grated lime zest

¼ cup lime juice

2 tablespoons finely chopped palm sugar, or packed brown sugar (see Tip)

2 tablespoons fish sauce

Hawaiian chiles, or any fresh hot chiles, minced, to taste

3 cups matchstick-cut or julienned green papaya, (see Tip)

½ cup very thinly sliced Maui or other sweet onion

½ cup pea shoots, cut into 3-inch pieces, or bean sprouts

Freshly ground pepper, to taste

Directions

Step 1

Whisk lime zest, lime juice, sugar, fish sauce and chiles in a large bowl.

Step 2

Add papaya, onion and pea shoots (or sprouts) to the vinaigrette; toss to combine. Sprinkle with pepper just before serving.

Tips

Make Ahead Tip: The vinaigrette (Step 1) will keep, covered, in the refrigerator for up to 1 week.

Palm sugar is an unrefined sweetener similar in flavor to brown sugar. It's sold in "pods" or as a paste in Asian markets or at importfood.com.

Nutrition Facts
Serving Size: 2/3 Cup

Per Serving:

55 calories; 0.2 g total fat; 0.1 g saturated fat; 403 mg sodium. 141 mg potassium; 13.3 g carbohydrates; 1.3 g fiber; 9 g sugar; 1.4 g protein; 470 IU vitamin a iu; 36 mg vitamin c; 27 mcg folate; 19 mg calcium; 15 mg magnesium; 4 g added sugar;

Thai Pumpkin Soup

Ingredients

2 tablespoons red curry paste

4 cups chicken or vegetable broth about 32 ounces

2 15 ounce cans pumpkin puree

1 3/4 cup coconut milk or a 13.5 ounce can, reserving 1 tablespoon

1 large red chili pepper sliced

Cilantro for garnish if desired

Instructions

In a large saucepan over medium heat, cook the curry paste for about one minute or until paste becomes fragrant. Add the broth and the pumpkin and stir.

Cook for about 3 minutes or until soup starts to bubble. Add the coconut milk and cook until hot, about 3 minutes.

Ladle into bowls and garnish with a drizzle of the reserved coconut milk and sliced red chilis. Garnish with cilantro leaves if desired.

Mediterranean Tuna Salad

SERVES 2

Ingredients

2, 5oz cans tuna packed in water, drained

1/4 cup mayonnaise

1/4 cup chopped kalamata or mixed olives

2 Tablespoons minced red onion

2 Tablespoons chopped fire roasted red peppers

2 Tablespoons chopped fresh basil

1 Tablespoon capers

1 Tablespoon fresh lemon juice

Salt and pepper

2 large vine-ripened tomatoes

Directions

Add all ingredients except tomatoes in a large bowl then stir to combine. Slice tomatoes into sixths, without cutting all the way through, then gently pry open. Scoop Mediterranean Tuna Salad mixture into the center then serve.

Notes

Could also serve tuna salad as a sandwich, in a pita pocket, on a bed of greens, or with crackers.

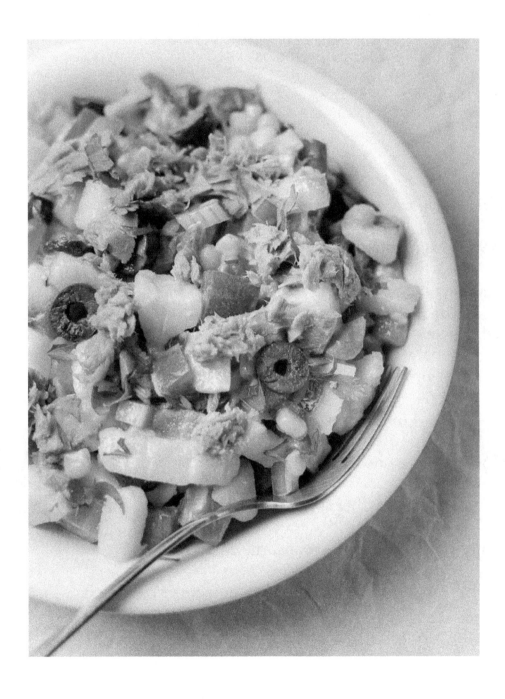

Slow Cooker Turkey Chili

PREP TIME 10 minutes

COOK TIME 4 hours

TOTAL TIME 4 hours 10 minutes

SERVINGS 8

Ingredients

1 tablespoon olive oil

1 lb 99% lean ground turkey

1 medium onion diced

1 red pepper chopped

1 yellow pepper chopped

2 (15 oz) cans tomato sauce

2 (15 oz) cans petite diced tomatoes

2 (15 oz) cans black beans, rinsed and drained

2 (15 oz) cans red kidney beans, rinsed and drained

1 (16 oz) jar deli-sliced tamed jalapeno peppers, drained

1 cup frozen corn

2 tablespoons chili powder

1 tablespoon cumin

Salt and black pepper to taste

Optional toppings: green onions shredded cheese, avocado, sour cream/Greek yogurt

Instructions

Heat the oil in a skillet over medium heat. Place turkey in the skillet, and cook until brown. Pour turkey into slow cooker.

Add the onion, peppers, tomato sauce, diced tomatoes, beans, jalapeños, corn, chili powder, and cumin. Stir and season with salt and pepper.

Cover and cook on High for 4 hours or low for 6 hours. Serve with toppings, if desired.

Note-we use a 6 quart slow cooker.

GINGERBREAD OATMEAL RECIPE:

Prep Time 5 mins

Cook Time 30 mins

Total Time 35 mins

Yield: 4 servings

Calories: 175 kcal

Ingredients

4 cups water

1 cup steel cut oats

1 1/2 tbsp. ground cinnamon

1/4 tsp. ground coriander

1/4 tsp. ground cloves

1/4 tsp. ground ginger

1/4 tsp. ground allspice

1/8 tsp. ground nutmeg

1/4 tsp. ground cardamom

Maple syrup to taste

Instructions

Cook the oats to package directions but include the spices when you add the oats to the water.

When finished cooking, add maple syrup to taste.

Recipe Notes

Please note that the nutrition data below is a ballpark figure. Exact data is not possible. Data below does not include maple syrup.

Nutrition Facts

Calories 175 Calories from Fat 27

% Daily Value*

Fat 3g 5%

Sodium 17mg 1%

Potassium 50mg 1%

Carbohydrates 32g 11%

Fiber 7g 29%

Protein 6g 12%

Vitamin A 35IU 1%

Vitamin C 2mg 2%

Calcium 95mg 10%

Iron 2.4mg 13%

* Percent Daily Values are based on a 2000 calorie diet.

Kale Cesar Salad with Grilled Chicken Wrap

Preparation time: 10 minute(s)

Number of servings (yield): 2

Ingredients

-8 ounces grilled chicken, thinly sliced

-6 cups curly kale, cut into bite sized pieces

-1 cup cherry tomatoes, quartered

-3/4 cup finely shredded Parmesan cheese

-½ coddled egg (cooked about 1 minute)

-1 clove garlic, minced

-1/2 teaspoon Dijon mustard

-1 teaspoon honey or agave

-1/8 cup fresh lemon juice

-1/8 cup olive oil

-Kosher salt and freshly ground black pepper

-2 Lavash flat breads or two large tortillas

Instructions

1. In a bowl, mix together the half of a coddled egg, minced garlic, mustard, honey, lemon juice and olive oil. Whisk until you have formed a dressing. Season to taste with salt and pepper.

2. Add the kale, chicken and cherry tomatoes and toss to coat with the dressing and ¼ cup of the shredded parmesan.

3. Spread out the two lavash flatbreads. Evenly distribute the salad over the two wraps and sprinkle each with ¼ cup of parmesan.

4. Roll up the wraps and slice in half. Eat immediately

THE BAKED TILAPIA RECIPE:

Prep Time: 15 minutes Cook Time: 18 minutes Total Time: 33 minutes Servings: 4 Servings Calories: 222.4kcal

Ingredients

1/3 cup chopped raw pecans

1/3 cup whole wheat panko breadcrumbs

2 teaspoons chopped fresh rosemary

1/2 teaspoon coconut palm sugar or brown sugar

1/8 teaspoon salt

1 pinch cayenne pepper

1 1/2 teaspoon olive oil

1 egg white

4 4 ounces each tilapia fillets

Instructions

Preheat oven to 350 degrees F.

In a small baking dish, stir together pecans, breadcrumbs, rosemary, coconut palm sugar, salt and cayenne pepper. Add the olive oil and toss to coat the pecan mixture.

Bake until the pecan mixture is light golden brown, 7 to 8 minutes.

Increase the heat to 400 degrees F. Coat a large glass baking dish with cooking spray.

In a shallow dish, whisk the egg white. Working with one tilapia at a time, dip the fish in the egg white and then the pecan mixture, lightly coating each side. Place the fillets in the prepared baking dish.

Press the remaining pecan mixture into the top of the tilapia fillets.

Bake until the tilapia is just cooked through, about 10 minutes. Serve.

Nutrition

Serving: 1Tilapia Fillet | Calories: 222.4kcal | Carbohydrates: 6.7g | Protein: 26.8g | Fat: 10.8g | Saturated Fat: 1.4g | Cholesterol: 55mg | Sodium: 153.3mg | Fiber: 1.6g | Sugar: 0.4g

WINTER FRUIT SALAD WITH PERSIMMONS, PEARS, GRAPES, AND PECANS

yield: 6 SIDE-DISH SERVINGS total time: 25 MINUTES prep time: 25 MINUTES

INGREDIENTS:

4 Fuyu persimmons, cut in 1 inch cubes (or enough cut persimmons to make 2 cups)

3 Bosch pears, cut in 1 inch cubes (or enough cut pears to make 2 cups)

1 cup grapes, cut into halves or fourths if large (I would have used more grapes if I'd had more)

3/4 cup pecans, cut into half lengthwise to make slivers

DRESSING INGREDIENTS:

1 T extra virgin olive oil (use a fruity oil for this)

1 T peanut oil

1 T pomegranate-flavored vinegar (I used pomegranate-flavored red wine vinegar)

2 T agave nectar or sweetener of your choice (If you have pomegranate molasses I might use white balsamic vinegar and substitute pomegranate molasses for some or all of the agave nectar)

Pinch of salt, to taste

DIRECTIONS:

Whisk together the dressing ingredients so flavors can blend while you cut the fruit.

Cut grapes, persimmons, and pears into same size pieces (about 1 inch size) and place in plastic bowl.

Toss fruit with dressing. Just before serving, toss with pecan pieces.

NOTES:

Other fruits such as apples, figs, or pomegranate arils could be used to replace any of these, but you need 5-6 cups of cut fruit.

Roasted Red Pepper and Sweet Potato Soup

Prep Time: 25 minutes Cook Time: 30 minutes Total Time: 55 minutes Yield: 6 servings

Ingredients

2 tablespoons olive oil

2 medium onions, chopped

1 jar (12 oz) roasted red peppers, chopped, liquid reserved

1 can (4 oz) diced green chiles

2 teaspoons ground cumin

1 teaspoon salt

1 teaspoon ground coriander

3 – 4 cups peeled, cubed sweet potatoes

4 cups vegetable broth

2 tablespoons minced fresh cilantro

1 tablespoon lemon juice

4 oz cream cheese, cubed

Instructions

In a large soup pot or Dutch oven, heat the olive oil over medium-high heat. Add the onion and cook until soft. Add in the red peppers, green chiles, cumin, salt and coriander. Cook for 1-2 minutes.

Stir in the reserved juice from the roasted red peppers, sweet potatoes and vegetable broth. Bring to a boil, then reduce heat and cover. Cook until the potatoes are tender, 10-15 minutes. Stir in the cilantro and lemon juice. Let the soup cool slightly.

Place half of the soup into a blender along with the cream cheese. Process until smooth, then add back into the soup pot and heat through. Season with additional salt, if needed.

ONE PAN LEMON HERB SALMON AND ZUCCHINI

Yield: 4 SERVINGS prep time: 15 MINUTES cook time: 20 MINUTES total time: 35 MINUTES

INGREDIENTS:

4 zucchini, chopped

2 tablespoons olive oil

Kosher salt and freshly ground black pepper, to taste

FOR THE SALMON

2 tablespoons brown sugar, packed

2 tablespoons freshly squeezed lemon juice

1 tablespoon Dijon mustard

2 cloves garlic, minced

1/2 teaspoon dried dill

1/2 teaspoon dried oregano

1/4 teaspoon dried thyme

1/4 teaspoon dried rosemary

Kosher salt and freshly ground black pepper, to taste

4 (5-ounce) salmon fillets

2 tablespoons chopped fresh parsley leaves

DIRECTIONS:

Preheat oven to 400 degrees F. Lightly oil a baking sheet or coat with nonstick spray.

In a small bowl, whisk together brown sugar, lemon juice, Dijon, garlic, dill, oregano, thyme and rosemary; season with salt and pepper, to taste. Set aside.

Place zucchini in a single layer onto the prepared baking sheet. Drizzle with olive oil and season with salt and pepper, to taste. Add salmon in a single layer and brush each salmon filet with herb mixture.

Place into oven and cook until the fish flakes easily with a fork, about 16-18 minutes.

Serve immediately, garnished with parsley, if desired.

Smoked Salmon Potato Tartine

YIELD: 2 SERVINGS

Prep time: 25 MINUTES

Cook time: 20 MINUTES

Total time: 45 MINUTES

INGREDIENTS
POTATO TARTINE:

1 large russet potato, peeled and grated lengthwise

2 tablespoons clarified butter (or other neutral flavored oil)

Kosher salt

Freshly ground black pepper

TOPPINGS:

4 ounces soft goat cheese, at room temperature

1 1/2 tablespoons finely minced chives

1/2 garlic clove, finely minced

Zest of half a lemon

Thinly sliced smoked salmon

2 tablespoons drained capers

2 tablespoons finely chopped red onion

1/2 hard-boiled egg, finely chopped

Finely minced chives (for garnish)

INSTRUCTIONS

Assemble Toppings: Combine goat cheese, lemon zest, and garlic in small bowl. Season with salt and pepper to taste. Gently stir in fresh chives. Set aside.

Season the chopped red onion and hard-boiled egg with salt.

Prepare Potato Tartine: Working quickly (as the potato will quickly begin to oxidize), grate the potato (lengthwise) into a large using the large holes of a grater. Squeeze the potatoes over the sink to remove any excess liquid. Season generously with salt and pepper and toss.

Heat clarified butter in a 8-10 inch non-stick skillet over medium-high heat. Once hot, add the grated potato and shape roughly, using a spatula, into a large circle.

Press on the mixture with the back of a spoon to compact it, cover and cook gently for 8-10 minutes or until the bottom is golden brown.

Flip carefully to other side and cook for another 8-10 minutes or until golden brown and crispy.

Remove to cooling rack and allow to cool until barely lukewarm or room temperature.

Assemble Tartine: Once potato cake has cooled, spread the goat cheese mixture on the top. Layer the smoked salmon directly over this and sprinkle with the red onion, hard-boiled egg, and capers. Garnish with freshly chopped chives. Cut into wedges and serve immediately.

NUTRITION INFORMATION:
Yield: 2 Serving Size: 1

Amount Per Serving: Calories: 496Total Fat: 28gSaturated Fat: 17gTrans Fat: 0gUnsaturated Fat: 9gCholesterol: 115mgSodium: 1641mgCarbohydrates: 37gFiber: 5gSugar: 3gProtein: 25g

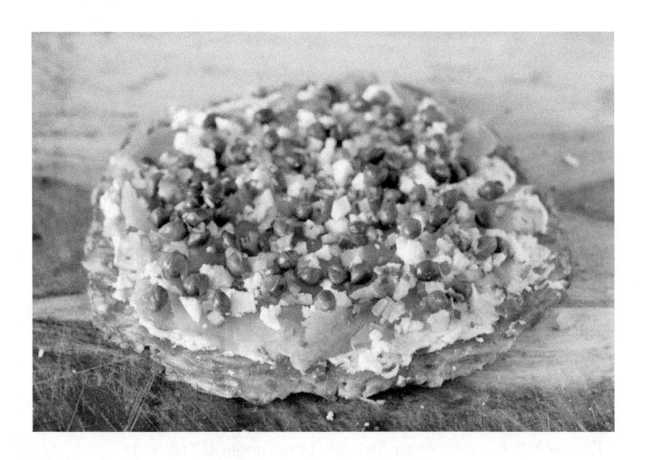

Red Lentil and Squash Curry Stew

Yield: ~4 servings

Ingredients:

1 tsp. extra virgin olive oil

1 sweet onion, chopped

3 garlic cloves, minced

1 tbsp. good quality curry powder (or more to taste)

1 carton broth (4 cups) I used low-sodium

1 cup red lentils

3 cups cooked butternut squash

1 cup greens of choice

Fresh grated ginger, to taste (optional)

Kosher salt & black pepper, to taste (I used about 1/2 tsp salt)

Directions

1. In a large pot, add EVOO and chopped onion and minced garlic. Sautee for about 5 minutes over low-medium heat.

2. Stir in curry powder and cook another couple minutes. Add broth and lentils and bring to a boil. Reduce heat and cook for 10 minutes.

3. Stir in cooked butternut squash and greens of choice. Cook over medium heat for about 5-8 minutes. Season with salt, pepper, and add some freshly grated ginger to taste.

Note: If you have uncooked butternut to use, check out Martha's recipe for cooking instructions.

Turkey & Quinoa Stuffed Peppers

Ingredients:

3 large yellow peppers

1.25lb extra lean ground turkey

1 C diced mushrooms

1/4 C diced sweet onion

1 C chopped fresh spinach

2 teaspoons minced garlic

1 C (1 8oz can) tomato sauce

1 C chicken broth

1 C dry quinoa

Directions:

In a small saucepan, start the quinoa and cook according to package directions (usually about 15 minutes).

While the quinoa cooks, saute the vegetables in a pan with a little butter or olive oil.

Then after about 5 minutes or so, add the ground turkey and garlic to the vegetables. Cook over medium heat. Once the turkey is mostly cooked though, add in the tomato sauce and about half of the chicken broth. Let simmer until the turkey is fully cooked and some of the excess liquid has cooked off.

Preheat the oven to 400.

While the turkey mixture simmers, prep your bell peppers. Wash the peppers, cut them in half, and remove the stem & seeds. Spray a 9×13 baking pan with cooking spray and place the cut bell peppers in the pan (open side up).

Once the quinoa is done cooking, dump it into the pan with the turkey & vegetables. Stir together. Then, stuff each bell pepper with the mixture. Make sure they are nice & full! If you're opting for cheese, then top with just enough cheese to barely cover the mixture (if you put too much on, it will get super messy in the oven!). Pour the rest of the chicken broth into the base of the pan (so around the peppers, not over them).turkey & quinoa stuffed yellow peppers

Cover with foil and bake at 400 for about 30-35 minutes. Serve warm & eat up!

Chapter three

Conclusion

People with RA may benefit from following an anti-inflammatory diet. Many recipes are available for each type of meal to help people follow this diet.

Anti-inflammatory diets are often healthful diets that promote healthy digestion and are usually free from harmful sources of fats, such as trans fatty acids. Instead, these diets contain healthful fat sources, such as fish and olive oil.

A person should always consult a doctor before starting a new diet or trying a supplement for the first time. These dietary changes can sometimes lead to negative interactions with medications or have an adverse effect on overall health.

CPSIA information can be obtained
at www.ICGtesting.com
Printed in the USA
BVHW011706210521
607866BV00013B/2466